"Dedicated to

the Health of my Country"

Walter M. Bortz, MD

OCCUPY MEDICINE

A Call For A Revolution

To Save American Health Care

TABLE OF CONTENTS:

A Mandate Mandate

Crisis creates opportunity. While the furor of the US Supreme Court mandate decision focuses on access and cost these are only tangential to the imperative issue which defines our broken health-care system.

Ours is not a Health-care system.
It is a Disease-care system.

It is a system in which all resources are consumed by repair. Repair is a fiscal and scientific black hole with a reciprocal connection between cost and benefit.

All the kings horses and all the kings men cannot make America healthy until it embraces a Commonhealth. A system in which every segment of society is committed to the assurance of our personal and collective potential. This is unarguably our most important national resource.

Assumption of individual responsibility is paramount.

Each of us owns our health. We cannot download it on government or doctors or pills.

The solution is a massive campaign to eradicate health illiteracy:

We need health in our classrooms and homes. Not expensive body shops.

Today we know enough to prevent 50 % of illness and save trillions of dollars.

Mean spirited and selfish short term political posturing demeans our nation's reach to full lives for all Americans.

Carpe Diem!

TAKE CONTROL OF YOUR HEALTH

Medicine wants you to be sick. The sicker you are, the more the medical corporation banks. It doesn't want you to be well and healthy. It doesn't want you to watch your diet and exercise and practice prevention. Prevention means healthy people. Healthy people don't need pills and procedures and hospitalizations and surgeries. Healthy people don't have diabetes and heart disease. So healthy people don't pay big medical bills. And without those big bills Big Medicine can't feed itself.

The Medical Monster needs to feed.

On You.

It's not a pretty picture.

But it's the Truth.

The only solution is a Revolution. The first steps toward that Revolution in American Medicine are information and knowledge. Only in recognizing this can we move forward and make change happen.

Occupy Medicine is a layman's handbook that hopes to guide you through the labyrinth of our present Medical Catastrophe.

American Medicine has morphed into a bureaucratic industrial complex whose core is the perpetuation of sickness.

Currently under intense political debate is the mandatory insurance coverage issue which is the central strut of Obamacare. America is the only civilized nation that doesn't have universal coverage.

Coverage of what?

Coverage of more CT Scans and dangerous drugs, excessive superspecialization, a doctor for every freckle and a procedure for every burp or fart?

Generations of Americans have voted for politicians who have been diffident and totally calloused to the common good. "Of, By, and For the People" has morphed into "For Me".

At age 82 I have enough wear on my tires, enough creases in my brow to audition these ideas for your consideration.

I believe myself to be as credentialed as any one else in the field of medicine and science speaking about this subject. I was Former President of the American Geriatrics Society, Co-Chairman of the AMA's Task Force on Aging and Clinical Professor of Medicine at Stanford.

I have 150 peer reviewed articles in the scientific literature, including JAMA and the New England Journal of Medicine. My father was President of the American Medical Association. I've authored seven books, have run a marathon a year for forty-one consecutive years and have nine grandchildren.

The material for this book is gathered from many sources. Paul Starr's sentinel work, "The Social Transformation of American Medicine" notes "its fall from sovereignty". Steve Schroeder, the esteemed past president of the Robert Wood Johnson Foundation, and now professor of medicine at UCSF asks pointedly "has medicine, lost its soul?"

Forces need to unite.

And those forces need information.

In order to look forward we must first look back:

It is widely suggested that the current outpouring of energy, which feeds the worldwide Occupy restlessness, has its origin in the Middle East, where governments are challenged as a result of the release of centuries of pent-up frustrations. Appeasement is being overthrown, the people speak loudly.

Why not us? If THEY can do it, why can't we? The French and American Revolutions and Egypt and Libya, etc sought liberty. Occupy Wall Street addresses too much liberty. According to Paul Krugman et al, the Wall Street outrage is the culmination of the rejection of this consummate greed.

Like other malignancies it spreads if it is not confronted.

REPLACEMENT PARADIGM

The drums are beating from far and wide.

We need a Revolution

In order for that to happen we need two things: First there must be agreement among the aggrieved parties that things are bad and that further appeasement is no longer an option. Second, and MORE important, there must be a Replacement Paradigm for the failed system.

There's no question that Medicine is suffering mightily on all fronts. Further agreement on this issue is not necessary. Young, old, north, south, labor, business, Republican, Democrat. We all agree that one of the central struts of our nation is crumbling. What has been lacking for the success of a Revolution in Medicine until now has been the replacement paradigm.

I contend that this replacement is at hand. This new paradigm is now scientifically enabled because we now understand WHAT HEALTH IS.

Up until now we have spent all of our intellectual and financial reserves on defining disease, because that's where the money is. Nobody notices when things go right. Health for a person is like water to a fish, a presumption. It is for this reason that health has been underappreciated and securely under-funded.

OCCUPY !

The largest single cause of personal bankruptcy in the US is health-care costs. Almost silently the medical care system has ridden the lack of oversight on the coattails of big money. A long look into the rearview mirror of Medicine reveals what was once a storefront operation of modest claim on societal resources has evolved into the voracious medical black hole.

The appetite of what is now the nation's biggest business is huge. Executives holding the big levers and manipulating the ledger sheets ride their corporate jets above the motley crowd.

The 99%.

Corporations lose competitive advantage not due to inferior product, but because they can't pay the hospital bills of their workers. They move overseas where it is cheaper to be sick.

The distress caused by this medical mess is only a part of the general sense of disenfranchisement and hopelessness. Despite our nation's extravagant GDP, its distribution across the populace is nearly at the bottom.

This misdistribution has occurred largely in the last 10 years and has immensely contributed to the sense of disenfranchisement. Exploitation gives rise to frustration.

Politicians and bankers are comfortable targets of our national distress, but what about doctors and nurses? They are here to take care of us, even if we can't do it ourselves. Yet their status as one of the central struts of our nation has been corrupted by their infrastructure.

My message is that:
It's not the doctors and nurses.

It's not the hospital administrators and their medical "bean counters".

It's not Big Business.

Not Big Government.

It's not the Democrats.

It's not the Republicans.

It's not Bill Maher.

It's not Russ Limbaugh.

It's YOU.

You are the only one who can

TAKE BACK MEDICINE!

Chapter 1   Take Control

What is the most important asset in your life?

Who owns that asset?

It belongs to you!

Do you understand that your life and your body belong to YOU?

Are you so brainwashed or diminished that you believe otherwise?

It's time to take control of what's Yours.

For ten years I gave the first lecture at the prestigious Stanford Business School Summer Program. They used me as their kickoff man to get the crowd fired up. My audience was a combination of CEO's and CFO's from some of the most influential companies in the world who attended with the express hope of getting richer. I challenged these Titans of Industry with the following questions,

"What's your greatest asset?" and "Who owns it?"

This begins the debate I introduce:

Only YOU own your most precious asset, your health.

"YOU are the only one who Can and Must TAKE IT BACK!"

This heraldic cry for a Revolution in Medicine finds allies within the international demand for the overthrow of authoritarianism in all its forms. The Wall Street ferment arose with the great awakening against the outrageous greed which permeates our entire society. Our World.

We, the people, lost 9 million jobs and 12 trillion dollars of net worth as 18 billion dollars were diverted to executive bonuses and $700 billion to rescue the derelict banks. While the 99% passively looked on and our government fiddled, the fat cats smiled. Bernie et al made us all look foolish.

In his recent book, the Price of Civilization, Jeffrey Sachs, identifies four domains which are particularly egregious. Big Oil, Wall Street, the Military-Industrial Complex, and Big Medicine are the villains. The fact that Medicine is included in this grouping offends me mightily. Do you really mean that Big Medicine is in the company of these scoundrels? The excesses exacted by these monstrous power centers demean all of us and erode our national character.

Big Medicine is the largest and most powerful corporation in the nation. And the only one of this gang that is totally out of control. Its by-laws foment injustice.

Inequality of access and outcomes are flagrant. But they are only a minor disgrace. Far worse is the reality that Big Medicine forces us to buy the wrong product. Big Medicine sells Disease. It should sell Health. The pretense is that it is taking care of our well being. The reality is that it is taking care of its own well being, and thereby constituting the single cause of personal and national bankruptcy. Despite a cost that is a multiple that of all countries, even Slovenia, the USA ranks 50th in life expectancy and 45th in low birth weight babies.

A Bitter Pill.

Don't swallow!

Loss of trust in the physician. Greed and commercialism have contaminated the critical social role of the doctor. Professionalism has ceded its moral claim on society's confidence to the Corporation of Medicine. Despite a generous paycheck, most physicians wouldn't do it again. We must make Medicine a profession again.

The largest contributor to poor health, the Actual Cause of Death is lifestyle. Since irresponsible personal behavior is our principle pathology then we need a cataclysmic shift.
A shift that emphasizes behavioral medicine.

Touch replaces Tech.

The entering medical student today learns a new shorthand vocabulary LOL, LMD, LOC; little old lady, local medical doctor, and loss of consciousness.

I have used these thousands of times, but LOC now has an additional, more important meaning, which is Locus of Control. The Locus of Control is a fundamental fact of health. It is within us, not external. We must grapple it to our souls.

The bio-ethicist Mark Sigler of the University of Chicago has an urgent perspective on this. He traces the rapid evolution from the centuries held position of the Medical Doctor as God, to the time when we began to question authority.

Sigler points to this second opinion era of Ralph Nader in which the patient assumed the upper hand. But this patient autonomy era lasted for only a brief time until now. Now enters the third era when bureaucratic parsimony kicks in.

We have now come to the grim point when neither what the doctor or patient decides is urgently important is heeded. That's because it's not you or your doctor who decides what you might want and need. The bureaucrats are now calling the shots.

It's depressing. It's depressing because of the sense that this thing is just too big for any of us to try and affect or control any longer. Like the Titanic heading for the proverbial iceberg … Americans, sick AND healthy, are confronted by a health care industry that, at its core, signifies the gradual depersonalization of medical care.

To a large extent doctors and nurses, the workers in the field, are now just passive observers in the takeover of their Good Samaritan ethic. Unfortunately they too have become co-dependent on the tides of greed that sweep them along. Individual health and well-being have been subverted to quarterly stockholder reports.

Until very recently the church has owned health. Now Big Medicine presumes ownership. Both are trumped up claims.

YOU own your health.

Any pretense to the contrary is wrong.

Trying to download your well-being to an indifferent and profit centered agency is doomed.

Chapter 2   Capitalism vs Biology

A robber confronts Jack Benny, "Your wallet or your life?"

A long pause.

Jack, "I'm thinking it over".

How can our bodies compete with our pocketbooks? Would you rather have your health or your money? The answer should be simple yet we struggle with these choices every day. What we eat. What we drink. How and whether we exercise. Do we smoke? Are we overweight and eating that extra dessert? Is our cholesterol too high yet we can't resist that three egg omelet?

We can't resist because we can't. It is human nature.

And as we humans struggle with this impossible dilemma, so too do the systems that mandate the control of our behaviors.

My recent book Next Medicine lists the many symptoms which accompany this hurt:

1) **Cost**
2) **Injustice**
3) **Danger**
4) **Corruption**
5) **Inefficiency**
6) **Inconsistency**
7) **Irrelevance**

In seeking the diagnosis of this complex of symptoms, I conclude the overriding culprit is a fundamental mismatch between capitalism and biology.

The administrative structure we have chosen to address all of our daily dealings is capitalism. But capitalism itself is not the problem. The problem is the product that capitalism has chosen to sell. And it has made the WRONG choice.

Capitalism should sell Health instead of Disease.

Several years ago I was lecturing in Nashville, Tennessee to the first-year class at Meharry Medical School.

Meharry is important in that it is one of only two surviving predominantly black schools. A close colleague of mine there had invited me to give my traditional talk about successful aging, which is a common errand for me.

As I stood in the pit of the amphitheater I regarded my audience. It was a totally different collection than those in my first-year class 60 years before at the University of Pennsylvania. The audience before me now was black, they were young, south, they were female. I was old, white, north and male.

But it was not these major demographic differences that separated us so much as it was the twin features of knowledge and money.

Within the 60 years since my graduation, the medical text has expanded logarithmically.

Moore's Law is extravagantly exhibited. In my era we did not know about genes and how long we might live. The alpha and omega of life were obscure. We had just gotten antibiotics and insulin and were very inexpert in their use.

But an even bigger difference than knowledge between myself and my audience was money. In my student era, Medicine was a humble cottage industry consuming maybe 2% of our gross national product. Now it approaches 18%. My physician father was often paid by barter. I recall boxes of cherries and oil paintings being his payment. I can imagine confronting the Stanford Hospital accounting office with boxes of cherries and paintings to discharge any financial obligations there.

So acknowledging the immense demographic, knowledge, and financial gaps, we were extremely different. My audience was not me. I certainly was not they. Yet WHAM. it struck me, that despite these huge differences we were united compellingly by a devotion to the mission of our profession. Despite all of these differences the one binding commitment was a shared devotion to the MISSION of medicine.

As I said these words, I recognized their importance. But I was immediately confronted by the question of just WHAT is the mission of medicine after all?

What is medicine's job description?

After some stammering I proposed that the mission of medicine is THE ASSERTION AND ASSURANCE OF THE HUMAN POTENTIAL. I paused mid sentence, recognizing the profundity of this observation. I quickly captured this concise definition, and have used it extensively since.

THE MISSION OF MEDICINE IS THE ASSERTION AND ASSURANCE OF THE HUMAN POTENTIAL.

It is what inspired Hippocrates and Galen, It nourished Florence Nightingale and Pasteur. The shamans and lab scientists share the same work bench. It is the common goal that drives doctors past, present, and future forward. It is one of humanity's noblest creeds.

But if we accept the generic challenge of the assertion of this potential we must ALSO recognize how miserably the medical profession fails in the second part of its mission; to assure the human potential.

It spends immense resources in this dereliction.

It is a square peg and a round hole not meshing at all.

Chapter 3 Tipping Point

Our entire American culture is staggering under the weight of the multiple burdens created by this mismatch.

Our health is up for auction.

Bids are accepted with little concern for true value. Instead the highest bid prevails. SOLD TO THE HIGHEST BIDDER.

Our forefathers would recoil at the erosion of our national character. Our ferocity of accumulation of wealth places us on a hedonic treadmill. Consumerism has led to a disruption of the American democratic process. Political influence is bought, rather than earned.

We have squandered our virtue in the pursuit of wealth. We have lost our civic nobility.

Accordingly, the majority of current society has hunkered down. Our social immune system is compromised and procrastination allows the distress to go unaddressed. We ask how much pressure must there be before the dam breaks, or whenever the next step takes us over the cliff.

Where is the Tipping Point?

Physicists call this transition moment a phase transition, where water becomes steam. When the bubble bursts, and when the tipping point is exceeded. Even Jesus, confronting the money lenders in the temple reached a bursting point of tolerance. How much must we hurt before we cry "Ouch?"

We have allowed our distractions to obscure responsibility. We seem to be numbed by the complexity of our world and are lulled by too much of everything. Peace and contentment are scarce commodities as we seek for "more". When is more enough? Rockefeller noted "one more dollar." But numerous studies show that more income does NOT bring more life satisfaction or longer life.

Famed international economist Jeffery Sachs quotes, "Living doesn't cost much. Showing off does." Instead of the Golden Rule, Buddhist philosophy, and Kant's Categorical Imperative being our compasses, we have been captured by our capitalistic desire for more possessions. Everything is for sale.

Even our health.

Our civitas has been eroded by special interests.

Medicine has become a giant corporation, the Medical Industrial Complex instead of a profession.

We are providers and consumers, not real people. We have lost our collective responsibility. Consumerism has conquered our conscience.

Sachs's book meticulously details how the lack of self respect by our financial institutions led to a feeding frenzy and the worldwide discord of stupendous proportion.

Trust, whatever there was of it at the beginning, has been lost as we passively hope that the whole mess will simply go away.

When tolerance is exceeded, we too easily lapse into circumstances where the moneylenders are appeased instead of evicted. Further accommodation is no longer possible. It demands address. The lobbyists create a corporatocracy. Self policing is random and ineffective. Distrust incurs disengagement.

The collective, the Common Cause, languishes. The defense of the Common Man becomes subverted to special interests.

We have become a nation of strangers.

The economic hubris of our corporate executives who continue to plunder is obscene. Sachs particularly labels the loss of compassion as a cardinal symptom of our time. We suffer from a collective anxiety of meaninglessness.

Our manifest inequality in capital and income distorts all. The rich get richer. The poor become poorer and the cascade leads to progressive poverty for all.

It is clear that central to all this unease lies our abandonment of social responsibility. We have become cynical, pessimistic and distrustful. Americans have always been wary of our governance, but now this lack of allegiance to anything that smacks of authority is hurtful to all.

We resent oversight and regulations, but this abandonment has allowed the benign problems of yesterday to become the spreading malignancy of today.

Are we better off than yesterday?

Our mission now is to occupy today.

And tomorrow.

And tomorrow.

Chapter 4 Redefining Medicine

Is medicine about health or disease?

Is medicine about function or dysfunction?

Is medicine about repair or prevention?

Health gets no respect, it is too implicit, like water is to a fish. We all know Zimmerman's law: people don't notice when things go right.

How about paying for health, not disease?

How about having incentives for health?

Now that we have the true metrics of health, its space and pace and span why don't we use this wonderful new knowledge to encourage people and medicine to move toward a "Health Model"?

Revisit the HMO.

We are now able to write a specific equation for health with defined exponentials. We now know the determinants of health. And it's the same as the determinants of your car's health; design, age, maintenance, accidents.

Mr. Aristotle got it right, the whole is much more than the sum of its parts. We know more and more about less and less.10 medical specialists don't equal one general practitioner.

Which floor of the enterprise am I on? Am I on the heart floor or the kidney floor or the ovary floor or the whole person floor?

What about me, all of me? We need whole people doctors, not parts of people doctors.

Chapter 5 Use it or Lose it

Not trite or trivial, but cosmic.

A profound TRUTH.

Why is exercise good for everything? Why is inactivity bad for everything? We were born to move for our food, but are now "Zoo Animals". We sit passively behind the zoo cage bars munching on Big Macs and fries. Our physiology requires that we are out running around hunting for food, gathering. Not sitting getting fat eating junk.

Domestication is bad for vitality. Activity is the universal prescription. It's readily available, safe, cheap and effective. Imagine if we could put it in a capsule, or in our drinking water?

You become what you do.
When you don't, you aren't.

We are flexible, elastic, constantly remaking ourselves in response to environmental signals.
Nature abhors stagnation. Exercise is a 30 year offset. A fit person of 70 is the same as an unfit person of 40. It's got nothing to do with doctors or pills or heredity. It's all about just getting up and USING our bodies the way they were designed to be used ten thousand generations ago.

VO2 Max: Sounds complicated but it simply means the transport of oxygen through our bodies. It's simple but it's our most critical function.
We don't do well without oxygen.

The disuse syndrome: Cardiovascular vulnerability, musculoskeletal fragility, metabolic instability, nervous system liability, immunological susceptibility, and precocious aging (frailty); all are secondary to a maladaptive lifestyle.

How many different doctors will I need to take care of my disused organs?

What does this disuse look like …. What does it do to me over time?

Diabetes, congestive heart failure, coronary heart disease, obesity, fractured hip, breast cancer, depression, progressive cultural inactivity.

Electric tooth brush, carving knife, TV clicker, golf cart (That's the worst!)

Bones, muscles, arteries, membranes, enzymes, brains all need to be used or they shrivel.

The Medicare Drug Entitlement Bill? My testimony against it:

Be an exclamation point, not a comma!

Look at the relationship between exercise and Alzheimer's Disease; BNDF is brain derived neurotrophic factor. It's Miracle Grow for the brain and it GOES UP with exercise.

Take a walk and not a pill!

Chapter 6   The Hurtful Gene

Over promised and under delivered.

Naïve, dangerous, corrupt, stupid, tragic these adjectives characterize the route that medical science has been on for the past several decades. It has been nourished by commercial obsession, but it has been wrong. The promise of great prestige and great wealth dangled. Pursuit of the gene has cost us several decades and several treasuries full of progress.

The history of scientific endeavor is characterized by reductionism, taking things apart to see how they work.

The epitome of this is the gene.

When I was in medical school we did not even know there was such a thing. All of a sudden it became the Holy Grail, which, when we conquered it, would give us all the answers as to who we are or might be.

Just because we've taken it down to the smallest particle does not yield much understanding. Is smaller better?

The Selfish Gene.
"My Genes made me do it".

Genocentrism has distorted our biologic reality. We become what we do.

We are constantly remaking ourselves in accord with our environment. Genes are miniature switches that are like rheostats, which are intimately cued. Not just off and on, but precisely susceptible to the messages which the environment provides.

We are different at different times. Our atoms are 98% different each year. We are the 2012 edition of ourselves not the 2011 or 2013. We are fantastically plastic. This critical reality is unrecognized by modern medicine, which presumes constancy but the facts speak dynamics.

There is no stasis in life. All life is dynamic, our brains, our arteries, our bones, ourselves are direct byproducts of choices we make daily and don't make.
Who we are is what we do.
When we don't we aren't.

The auditorium was packed in anticipation of Nobel Laureate Arthur Kornberg's full elaboration of the human genome; Huge Moment in the History of Science.!! Greah Hurrah's. I raised my hand and said, "I don't see genes in my practice, what I see is behavior" but I do not see behavior celebrated in the journals.

He replied "that is because there is no science in behavior". I was immediately embarrassed for him, but his fixation made the point of how far big science has strayed from the truth.

The buzz term these days is personalized medicine. This public relations term is really a repackaging of the failed model of the gene. For all it's overpromising it does occasionally contain value although much less than it pretends.

Personalized medicine is depersonalized medicine. Neglect of the effect of our nurture on our nature pretends that our destiny is coded before us. Wrong dangerously wrong.

GWAS EWAS

GWAS stands for Genome Wide Association Studies and is the inclusive term for the many thousands of experiments done and papers written seeking to establish the genetic basis of compulsive gambling, freckles, and hosts of other life irregularities.

GWAS has failed because of its neglect of the plasticity of the gene. It's not the cards you're dealt it's how you play the hand.

My Stanford gene expert friends recognize this and have amended GWAS to EWAS; Environment Wide Association Studies, in which the gene is placed in full context both spatially and temporally.

It is how life works.

This new perspective is vastly more complicated. It acknowledges the reality of the complexity and uncertainty, which, if not contained within the scientific mantra, makes a mockery of earlier claims for comprehensive knowledge.

My science buddies and I put on a meeting at the NIH ten years ago entitled the Dynamics and Energetics of Health and Aging. International experts congregated and spent three days advocating for a new emphasis beyond the gene on the SYSTEM rather than its components, on PROCESS rather than episode.

Collectively we wrote the Director of the NIH and encouraged him to shut the Gene Institute and emphasize the system and its behavioral components in a new System Institute. Instead and to our immense disappointment, he placed Francis Collins, the head of the Gene Institute as Director of the entire N.I.H.

We must wait a bit longer for the gene addiction to pass.

Chapter 7   Missing Touch

A GATHERING SORE

Ouch !

In just a few decades the medical system has convulsively transformed from a simple gentle cheap store-front operation to the largest industry in the world. Gone are the hand-written notes, the solo practice, the penlights, tongue depressors and stethoscopes of my youth ceded to the electronic robots which inhabit the cavernous canyons of today's repair industry and who are in instant touch with the accountants who monitor every possible billable item.

Like a deer caught in the headlights we are dazzled by the wizardry which is an alien world run by corporations, strangers. Along the way huge scientific insights into our most minute anatomy have emerged. Whole mountainsides of data are cached. We are fully dissected. The economic impact of this progressive ouch is profound and threatens the entire organism.

But what if the original cause of our ouch was a tiny splinter in a toe which did not yield awareness of its presence to high-priced specialists and technologies?

What if high tech is low touch, and touch is the missing tool?

It was Palm Sunday morning. We had arrived at the cavernous hall known as Howrah Train station in Calcutta. Having ridden the Madras Express up the east coast of India. The night before we had been submerged into the phantasmagoria of the Bubeneshwar religious Hindu festival with sense numbing cymbal crashes, horns blaring, immense juggernaut floats, smoke, incense, fireworks, screams. It was psychedelic in the extreme.

The subsequent efforts to sleep on the continuing train ride northward were restless. On an eerie predawn we were immediately swallowed into the swirl of Calcutta. After a quick cab trip to a nearby tourist hotel, we ventured onward.

We had in important errand to run.

Within an hour I had rung the small bell at the walled sanctuary, which was Mother Teresa's convent. I was ushered to a canopied table in a quiet courtyard. And there was Everyperson's Saint, Mother Teresa.

I presented my credentials. "Mother, I am an American physician who has made his life career the medical issues of older people, and am daily confronted with seemingly insoluble problems."

I described my several decades of medical practice seeking to serve as a caring steward of the downsides of my patients' lives, pondering and struggling with the uncertaincies and complexities of life's terminus.

Patiently she considered a moment and responded "Dr. Bortz, don't worry about all of that. Just love them." I hear her words as clearly now as they were at that moment.

"Just love them".

This simple advice left me speechless. Love was not in my list of internet search items. "Just love them", is not in the textbooks of my training as a physician.

I am sure that I must have shifted my position in my chair uneasily as I pondered her advice. She diffused my unease by offering, "Please come to my Home for the Dying tomorrow and perhaps you can learn from that".

Our visit probably lasted less than an hour. Mother Teresa certainly had other more important errands to run on this holy day, but her power for generosity of spirit has stayed with me ever since.

The following morning I went to her Home for the Dying. It was a nondescript medium-sized compound nearby and could easily be confused with a high school gym. One section was for males the other for females. Cement floors, wrought iron beds.

The young staff, mostly all volunteers wore green aprons. I donned mine and inserted myself unobtrusively into the scene. It was quiet, with gentle murmurs as the only conversation. Little medicines was available, The charts were only a few scribbles on a sheet.

Patients died, usually within several days. The women die of sepsis and the men from tuberculosis.. There was no aura of foreboding. The staff, Aussie, German, American, Indian was occupied with bathing and cleaning and feeding. I found myself sitting next to the bed of an emaciated woman who was barely conscious.

Awkwardly I entreated her to eat some of the porridge which I offered from my bowl, managing to get more on myself than into her mouth. I felt grossly incompetent and feeble as I tried to help by bringing dignity, comfort, and possibly love to this dying woman.

I emerged from my visit of several hours later into the hubbub of Calcutta, forever changed by the experience.

Upon return to Stanford my first Medical Grand Rounds was delivered by a colleague who was discoursing about the new elegant visualizing technique for the coronary arteries. With this procedure we are newly able to provide the operating surgeon with an accuracy of precision which extends down to 1 mm in depth.

"All we need for this new competence is a linear accelerator", which Stanford just happens to have just off campus up the hill.

All $3,000,000,000 of it.

It was a stunning moment and I sat bolt upright in my seat and said to myself, "The world has gone mad.

Mother Teresa doesn't have a pinch of penicillin or an ounce of anesthesia for her dozens of dying patients, but here we are at Stanford dealing with in a gilded technology of minor value.

The world has gone mad.

Several weeks later, I recorded this strange juxtaposition to Jim Wyngarden, who was then head of the NIH. He volunteered his similar discomfort when he signs his name to the granting of Mega millions of dollars to research projects dealing with such arcane topics as potassium transport in toad bladders. He similarly ponders whether such expenditure is appropriate with millions of our people lacking medical insurance and care.

Chapter 8   Ah Ha!

Every Wednesday morning, ritually almost without fail my day starts at 8 a.m. at the Grand Rounds at Stanford, where the Department of Medicine conducts its principal educational gathering. 300 seekers attend. Usually the presentation derives from a case of a patient who was recently encountered. The details of the case are described by the interns and residents who have been involved.

Three months ago the case was that of a young woman from the Caribbean who by some route arrived in the Stanford emergency room complaining of severe backache.

The initial evaluation revealed sufficient cause for the ER physician to arrange her admission to the medical floor of the hospital.

Corps of physicians of all persuasions descended. Sequences of lab tests were ordered, pints of blood were scrutinized, each corner of her body was scanned, several times. A variety of seemingly unconnected abnormalities were revealed. Her pain persisted. The patient's condition deteriorated. The aggregated findings became ever more complex and puzzling. The diagnosis remained obscure.

After several days of further sleuthing into the cause of the ouch a junior resident was called by a radiologist who asked, "What are you doing about the breast cancer?"

"What breast cancer?"

Among the scores of examinations that had been performed at Stanford Medical center's top echelon was a chest x-ray in the emergency room en route to admission to the hospital which showed a mass in the breast.

But the report had become lost in he avalanche of other subsequent more exotic tests. The diagnostic effort failed to trigger. Nowhere in the chart was there any mention of her breast ever having been examined by an examiner's hands.

This dereliction screams, but it is not rare. Common disease is increasingly obscured by the esoterica. The simple reason was the neglect of a primitive protocol.

This case actually prompted an op-ed piece in the New York Times by Dr.Abraham Verghese, pointing out that touch often supersedes tech and should never be relegated to a laboratory presumption.

Reaching deeper yet into what should have happened is the reality that the woman should have found the lump on her own, either because of enlightened self interest or because of regular prompts from a health reoriented medical system.

Chapter 9   Occupy Fat

Fat is not fate.

Fat is a choice.

Our children die before us. Theirs is the first generation to die before their parents because of fat. Half of the population of the US is fat.

Now we know enough to require obese people to be responsible.

A Fat Tax.

Charge by the pound.

Pay by the pound

It may sound outrageous but why should society "pay" for unhealthy behavior?

The economics of obesity.

Perhaps airlines should charge by the pound. Or how about redesign of Yankee Stadium to accommodate wider buts and charging more for them? The possibilities are endless.

The roots of fat: My 51st birthday was spent with a tribe on the Kalahari where my friendly hosts toasted me with "May all your children be fat".

We move to eat, we eat to move. All of our ancestors were athletes who ate what they could catch and avoided being eaten.

What is the right diet? For what amount of exercise?

Questions. Answers.

Upon my father's death I became a geriatrician. It was a transformative time. I moved from Philadelphia to California and started to run as a healing effort.

My new life as a runner immersed me in marathons and in the Western States 100 mile race, among the World's toughest endurance tests. I became fascinated in observing those fine athletes stress themselves to the fullest human potential. They would run for 24 hours straight up and down the steep canyons of the Sierra Foothills through temperatures ranging from freezing to 100 degrees. My son did it. My wife did it. I would crew for them and my amazement grew so much so that I decided to do an experiment on the Western States runners; I drew their blood at the finish line and initiated research on the runners' level of endorphins and measured the size of their arteries.

"Who cares what your cholesterol is if your artery is an inch across?"

Fitness covers up a lot of sinning.

Modern medicine is woefully inadequate to address this world wide Obesity epidemic; its twin tools of pharmacy and surgery are dangerous and possibly criminal. Surgery for obesity is similar to amputating the fingers of a smoker.

Fat is not Fate.
Fat is a Ghoice.

The choice is Yours.

Chapter 10   Occupy Dying

Woody Allen:" I'm not afraid of dying, but I don't want to be there when it happens."

A good death? No tubes, no pain, no loneliness.

What ever happened to a natural death? Expected, anticipated death. Death that involves a family gathering together around a loved one to comfort each other until the end.

Today we die poorly by bits and pieces, we die component deaths rather than system deaths.

We die too long.

The medical industrial complex now owns the death industry.

The home setting of the famous painting, "the Doctor", is now the tumult of the ICU, with robots tubes and accountants in attendance.

We now have death contingencies.

WHERE to die?

Increasingly we find ourselves dying in hospitals. This is certainly not a natural death.

Too many of us are in nursing homes.

The hospice movement.

Is euthanasia okay?

Geographic variance in cost of death, physicians profit from pursuing futility, do we prolong life or prolong dying?

WHEN to die?

My Granddaddy Bortz, his old advice is now life shaping for me:

Be Necessary.

Be a resource, not a liability.

What time is it in your life? Is it time to die or live? Live until you die.

Death is often a choice, Suicide Prevention statement "suicide is a permanent answer to an often temporary situation".

HOW to Die.

Dad's death, Mother's death.

Norman Cousins "accept the diagnosis but reject the verdict".

The solution to death anxiety is to live a long time.

Centenarians welcome death.

My vision of a Perfect Death for myself will happen as the ultimate beachcomber. I will be on a beach looking toward the west. As death approaches I will stop eating and drinking. As the sun sinks my carcass shuts down. I will lie on the sand and the waves will take me out.

 After Dying
No oblivion, ripples!

Immortality is mine, is for all of us. We live on in the lives of all whom we have touched.

Chapter 11 Flexner

ABRAHAM FLEXNER WE NEED YOU   AGAIN!

How many times do we get a second chance?

A chance to reformulate?

To resurrect. To renaissance.

Rebirth.

When such a rare opportunity presents there are only seconds before the flame is gone.

Those seconds are ticking.

Medicine is gasping for breath. It is cyanotic. But in order to save it by moving forward we must first look back. It was 100 years ago that Medicine gasped as well. And thanks to Abraham Flexner we did something about it and American Medicine came back to life.

100 years ago Medicine was in a dreadful state. Nearly anyone could become a doctor with nearly no credential. Any pretense of legitimacy was swamped by the realities of greed, incompetence, and ignorance. In 1875, Charles Elliot, President of Harvard University, wrote "the ignorance and general incompetency of the average graduate, at the time he receives a degree which turns him loose upon the community, is something horrible to contemplate".

Abraham Flexner, 1910, went on to overthrow medical education. Until then the payment of the faculty was from the students. Students could "buy" their MD. The majority of students enrolled without a college degree.

My Uncle Walter, for whom I was named, was admitted directly into Jefferson Medical College from high school in 1905.

Schools faced dire challenges to shape up, and thereby spend more money in the process, or hang on and pretend to be compliant, or fail. Flexner visited every one of the 155 medical schools in the country. He snooped widely, opening doors and drawers. He interviewed Deans and students and clerks.

Flexner's report was scathing. He found academic misrepresentations everywhere, especially between what was supposed to be a curriculum and what was learned. Originally he favored reduction in the number of schools to 31. However this stirred up such a ruckus that it eventually died.

Ultimately, Flexner's careful scrutiny resulted in the most momentous change in the history of American medicine.

That WAS THEN.

NOW IS NOW.

ANY DIFFERENCE?

It is now a full century since the original Flexner I of 1910 was mandated.

The perspective, "American Medical Education 100 years after the Flexner Report", was published recently in the New England Journal of Medicine by Cooke et al. It urges a reconfiguration of the "ossified curricular structures, the persistent focus on the factual minutiae of today's knowledge base, distracted and overcommitted teaching faculty, archaic assessment practices, and the abundance of historical constraints."

The authors comment that the current academic atmosphere is the result of faculty advancement being dependent mostly on research productivity rather than teaching, caring for patients, and the address of broader public health issues.

The hoped for result of a revisit of Flexner would be the graduation of an" informed, compassionate, curious, proficient and
moral physician."

I applaud this nomination.

The amount of financial commitment to health care in the Flexner I era was 2% of the GDP. Today it is 17%. Currently David Cutler of Harvard is steadfast in his insistence that this increase is not without merit. He would even allow it to go higher as part of a societal commitment.

Others are not so sure. Even if Cutler is correct that America is so rich that it can afford 20 or more percent of the GDP to fund the MIC, the propriety of this allocation calls for intense scrutiny.

In my first book, "We Live too Short and Die too Long", I created a graph that showed the increase in both the medical expense and knowledge over the last 80 years. I contrasted that with the gain in life expectancy of the average 40 year-old man which increased by eight years, compared with the virtually logarithmic increases in knowledge and dollars.

So what have we bought from this knowledge and expense? It is a modest return.

This embarrassment is made even worse by identification that life expectancy may be going down for the first time in our republic's history.

How can we be so rich and so smart and have so little to show for it?

.

Any educational change will require gross reworking of our network of laws and regulations, which now govern the practice of medicine.

Most of these have long outlived their moment and were constituted most to constrain competition as well assure quality.

Such curtailment of competition has squelched experimentation.

We must break out of the strictures. New systems of care and education will require new training protocols.

But of course, right there in the way is the huge issue of cost.

In the July 28, 2011 edition of the New York Times is an article by Dr. Paula Chan, which addresses the oppressive career, and indeed, societal effects of high training costs. Medical school tuitions approach $50,000. These changes mirror the US health expenditures which in 1960 were $863 per person per year. They were $8,855 per person per year in 2011.

Paying off student medical school debt sometimes takes decades. Over 80% of medical graduates are in debt, the average amount of which is $158,000, some extending well over $200,000 per person.

Such observations lead to an op-ed New York Times May 28, 2011 column by two health policy scholars, Peter Bach and Robert Koch. "Why medical schools should be free."

The under-valuing of primary care practice, which everyone except the specialists dare to identify as a central social wrong, is a paramount issue.

Removing the bondage of medical school debt would go far in reshaping the medical care work force of 15 million. If we could assure lower income equality it would show that civility can work.

LET US INITIATE A FLEXNER II

The multiple defects in medical education have upped the ante and make a re-examination, Flexner II, mandatory. If I were charged with arranging such a meaningful effort I would logically turn immediately to the medical school deans, the heads of departments at the NIH, the leaders of the drug and medical instrumentation companies, the American Hospital Association, the AMA, and other concerned entities.

I would turn them loose and say, "What do you see here one hundred years from now? What do you recommend for the next 100 years?"

I would be certain that this group of medical experts would effectively choose to clone their current enterprise. They are the fox guarding the hen house. The inmates would continue to run the asylum. What could one possibly expect from this 1% in their isolated ivory tower?

More and more of the same and the same.

But what if the same is wrong? Medicine now confronts an identity crisis that rivals that of 100 years ago. What if it's a square peg that doesn't fit the round hole as Abraham Flexner diagnosed a century ago?

Why can't we learn?

If this expert panel was franchised to search once again for medicine's soul it would have immense advantages over Flexner I.

We know incredibly more and spend incredibly more, to what benefit? My answer suggested above is, " to assure the human potential."

How much do we need to know to assure the human potential?

We need not know the approximate position of every electron or gene or red blood cell.

We DO need to know what the interplay of health determinants are to assure the potential of the organism.

Chapter 12   Problem or Solution?

Perhaps I am wishful in my suggestion, but it seems that the medical students themselves are likely to be the source of a reorientation of their training program. Professors are so committed and ingrained in their protocols they can only visualize a cloning of their success.

When placed against the default of fulfilling medicine's mission, one must call a spade a spade.

Currently I am involved with a group of 30 Stanford students who have created a new optional course on lifestyle medicine.

The course is specifically tailored on the model developed at Harvard by Dr. Eddie Philips. He has started the Harvard Lifestyle Medicine Institute, which I believe is game changing.

The course premise is around the curriculum called LIFE. It challenges medical students to address what the community needs ARE rather than an archaic relic which is no longer appropriate or relevant.

We need a square peg for a square hole. And we need a Flexner II with a blank slate that more accurately represents societal need. We now are awash in money and basic science, it is time to integrate these into the community health needs.

Illustrative of our local mismatch was a talk given to us doctors by the new director of the hospital, Amir Rubin. His first task in his exalted role is to preside over the $3 billion renovation of Stanford University Hospital that has languished in its earthquake susceptible buildings since the early Edward Stone creation 50 years ago.

As Rubin went through his show and tell he sketched broader and broader to boast of all the wizardry that will be in every corner. It will effectively be a huge ICU. The entire focus of the Silicon Valley mystique is to be extracted and inserted into what he proposes will be the hospital for the next 50 years. We attending doctors sat rapt with his projection of our future workplace.

I was restless.

At his conclusion, I raised my hand immediately and asked "what are you doing to keep people OUT of the hospital?"

An embarrassed hush was his response. But what kind of an answer did I expect? His responsibility is to the Stanford Board of Trustees, the 1% who expect black ink from their most expensive entity.

What can we expect from this?

Chapter 13 New World?

The global health needs now will not yield to technology. They are too personal. The consuming epidemic of chronic disease is grandly susceptible to prevention. With this stark, but only grudgingly acknowledged reality Next Medicine must INSIST on health rather than disease.

Flexner II must mandate that the WHOLE of Medicine become economically sound.

Health must pay.

The primary focus must be within the individual, not outside.

Behavior assumes highest priority.

Coming to grips with this insistency is deeply troubled by the fact that the mind and its behavioral secretions are denigrated. Tragically psychiatry's standing in the medical temple is deeply stained. Much of this stain was self-initiated.

Chapter 14   Behavioral Medicine

The principal villain in medical illness is the behavioral profile of the population. 65% of all chronic disease deaths and costs result from poor lifestyle. If lifestyle is the villain then it is critical that medicine target its research and training to this bull's eye.

Recall Arthur Kornberg's response to my contention that lifestyle was the 800 pound gorilla in my practice, hence it should lead medical pursuit. His reaction "there is no science in behavior" still echoes in my brain, because it reflected so powerfully on the disproportionate allocation within Big Science.

Behavior's seat in the pantheon of the NIH is almost invisible. "There is no science in behavior", hence no money.

This mismatch screams for redress.

A key On Common Ground effort was initiated in Kansas by Dr. Pat Deakin, herself a refugee from the chronic mental illness enclave. She has started a grass roots effort to ease the interface between the psychically needy and the understaffed mental-health system.

It is my firm feeling that if her effort can be cloned thousands of times it should relieve the dearth of trained persons. We cannot rely on people with advanced degrees exclusively to get us out of our collective mental funk.

As our mental health care system lags in the attention to mentally ill people, what about those of us who do not suffer illness but nonetheless are prisoners to adverse behaviors? There is so much work to be done taking care of not only the ill but those who by virtue of their self destructive behavior become ill that Flexner II must take a bright beam and shine it on this unmet domain.

Immediately adjacent to this frightening reality is that our friendly colleagues, the psychiatrists, the titular leaders of the behavior inquiry effort are in a crisis mode. Their entire world has been blitzed by their encounters with Big Pharma. It is no overstatement to observe that many if not most people now look at psychiatrists as whores for the pharmaceutical houses.

Our psychologic potential is a grand unknown. But with the arrival of a vastly expanded technology base mental health researchers' ability to generate a whole new curriculum of evidence-based science is a brilliant frontier.

Medicine's entire essence should be personal. Our godfather, William Osler, said "ask not what disease the patient has, but rather what patient has the disease. "The locus of control of medicine needs to go to the person rather than to the system. The system must address the human potential. Such a failed response to its job description is a huge demerit of our potential.

Our potential and its determinants are newly revealed, but they are imprisoned by the present self serving economic design. It is my sincere hope that the will of the people, the 99%, will demand that Medicine recapture its soul.

Chapter 15   Disruptive Prescription

Clayton Christiansen, prime mover of the Harvard Business School, speaks of the current medical mess in America as the 800-pound gorilla. Christiansen uses an industrial perspective in his assertion that, after all is said and done, medicine is large commerce. No morality, no romance allowed. It is a business and any effort to camouflage this reality is delusional.

I have long concluded that the solution to our medical distress will not yield to MDs, nurses, pharmacists or politicians, but must arise out of a business model.

Pragmatism is the only guide to progress.
Wishing is not going to make it happen.

Dollars will.

Christensen's book, the "Innovator's Prescription", proposes a large resorting of personnel, location, and regulations. He stresses that M.D and PhD advanced degrees are not necessary to treat the common cold, indeed are not necessary for 99% of every day needs. Practitioners are far overqualified for the work that they do.

Similarly he suggests that the primary sites of health care should be the home, school, and workplace rather than the hospital ICU, and operating rooms. His third major point concerns the regulatory changes, which will be necessary to effect personnel and location shifts.

These regulations are now archaic and often are remnants of the disheveled system in effect a century ago.

I personally endorse his prescription. It is my mantra of prevention over repair. Any Rx that facilitates this will serve us all brilliantly.

TOTAL BODY PAIN

Every facet of medicine today begs for a treatment. Service, education, research. All are stuck in a failed anachronistic model.

The primary service role which medicine has assumed is that of repair.

Instead, it should be prevention.

Its educational apparatus teaches new technology. It should address medical illiteracy.

Its research researches the wrong stuff. It targets components and episodes. It should focus instead on the whole and process. Its research agenda must realign to an understanding that the primary disease determinants of health are those of human behavior.

Different Staff:

Recognition of the value of lower level practitioners must be celebrated. The WHO has stressed the importance of self care. Development of primary care homes which intimately involve nurses, community pharmacists, and new resources even including dentists and telephone help lines extend the range of health care professionals. Available for common ailments and self-limiting illnesses and increased self-management is a prime consideration. The relation between home, office, clinic, hospital and ICU is blurred by new technology and different manpower.

I recall the immense gratification I felt when I hired the first nurse practitioner at the Palo Alto Clinic in the 1970s. Now there are dozens. The physician's assistant, the PA, and nurse practitioner, NP are close professional allies. A host of lower-level professionals have been repeatedly shown to produce actions and satisfactions which are equal to or greater than those of the MD.

Such activities have been grafted onto surgical specialties as well, as have office and home health-care responsibilities.

With this background, the Stanford Chronic Disease Self-Management Program was evolved. This has since morphed into what is known as the Expert Patient protocol. Thousands of persons worldwide have participated. The British National Health Service has embraced it as a central structure of their system. It has been translated into over 20 languages and is part of many national health programs.

In my view, we need an army of millions who will build the health efficacy of healthy people before they get sick. To prevent the need to repair is one of the principal goals of Occupy Medicine.

Different Venues?

Beyond the stretching of the physician's roll by the expanded use of allied paraprofessionals the tradition of the doctor's office as a first site of contact is being extended. In her November 27, 2011 column in the Wall Street Journal Market Watch Kristin Gerencher reports that visits to retail health clinics have jumped sharply.

In the November 2011 edition of the Journal of Managed Care she observes that the Rand Corp. studied retail clinics in pharmacies, shopping malls, and worksites and found that their use has expanded tenfold from 2007-2009.

These secondary outlets serve as an extension to provide care to those who find barriers in their standard site.

Walgreens has developed 400 such take care clinics; CVS pharmacy has developed medical clinics in more than half of the states. Walk-in medicine, drop in medicine, soon to be drive-through medicine emerge.

Such retail clinics are 30 to 40% cheaper than their similar rendered services in doctor's office, and 80 do 100% cheaper than visit to the hospital emergency room.

Urgent care clinics are similarly increasing. Beyond this extended range of care encounter zones the use of technology expands at every level of the care continuum from home to the ICU.

Telemedicine and Skype use by docs is expanding. If patients are able to talk with their kids using Skype why can' they do that with us? Some Stanford medical students are employing I pads to encourage the increased involvement of patients in the neighborhood health clinics.

Indeed self-monitoring of blood sugar, blood pressure, temperature, pulse rates, steps taken are new tools in medicine's black bag.

The hospital at home, HAH, is a protocol that is being evolved at Johns Hopkins, where individuals who present to the care system with a specified set of symptoms are shunted to a home care competence, which mimics that which would otherwise be provided when in hospital care. These are experimental and under extensive evaluation.

Expanding technology now involves instrumental diagnostic and therapeutic opportunities. Even to the suggestion of robotic surgery performed several continents away. These extensions now extend to the ICU where the e-ICU is in fashion. An article in the Boston Globe described the setting in Worcester Mass where an intensive care physician is working out of his office in a commercial building with an array of monitoring equipment in front of him. These were in turn connected to eight ICUs at hospitals in the University of Mass Memorial Hospitals, which involved 109 of their selected patients.

This arrangement of e-ICU was initiated because of insufficient supply of intensive care physicians. So they adopted a set of off-site units.

Talk about group practice!

Chapter 16   Commonhealth

All of the above is part of what I term a Commonwealth in which all segments of our society participate, not just the medical system, which has been shown to be not so large a determinant of our well-being as we all assume.

The medical health care complex is a necessary but insufficient component of the Commonwealth and only a minor part at that.

The hoped for impact the Commonwealth will have upon our system securely derives from:

I-O-I

Information, Opportunity, Incentive.

With this format I propose that Occupy Medicine has an organizing practical scheme to which we can ascribe:

I: Information

Wordsmiths tell us that the word "doctor" is derived from the Latin word decree to teach. David Cutler, Senior Professor at Harvard Business School, writes in a recent National Bureau of Economic Research publication, "effects of education on health and the probable reciprocal interchange".

Smart people live longer and better; have lower hospitalization rates, and lower pharmacy bills, fewer ER visits, healthier babies, on and on. Education policies have a substantial effect on health.

In 1999, death rates of high school dropouts were more than double those with some college education. One year of education equals .8 years of life lengthening. Both physical and psychological advantages accrue to people who are educated.

O: Opportunity.

Information is necessary but by itself insufficient. Knowledge needs the opportunity to be seen and heard and used. To impact this usage, it needs space and time. We need places to be healthy. Schools and workplaces are good places to start. Compulsory physical education within schools needs to be mandated, not an excuse. Work places need mandatory opportunities to move. The active desk is such a device seeking wider adoption. Parking lots should be placed at a distance. Stairs become the main route. Escalators and elevators are to be used only rarely.

And, of course, the biggest opportunity issue is time. "I don't have the time to be healthy" is the common lament.

Fast food, hurry illness are symptoms of our menaced use of time urgency.

I: Incentives

The last of the elements is incentives. Knowledge and opportunity need extra energy, which incentive supplies. Carrots and sticks.

Overall money is the BIG motivator.

There are manifest ongoing movements all over the country to search out the best ways of providing incentives. In my family, we adopted a program of rewarding our four children with $50 each if they didn't miss a day of school. They rarely if ever did.

The governor of Iowa boosts his state's role in the Blue Zones Healthy State Initiative boasting of the increased employment opportunities that accompany a healthier, and consequently cheaper workforce. The cost-benefit ratio of such programs is regularly affirmed to be somewhere in the range of three to seven to one.

I-O-I is an operational strategy that Occupy Medicine can use as a Disruptive Prescription.

The need is there.

The opportunity is here and now.

The know-how and incentives are in place.

Let us not let this time slip by.

Preach I-O-I.

Step up to the plate and OCCUPY!

Chapter 17 Answers?

We need a manifesto that matches need to system, a system that reflects what people NEED. Somebody said something about an America by, of, and for the people.

Really?

Our current medical corporation has no room for people.

Our patron saint Sir William Osler advised, "Seek not what disease the patient has, seek what patient has the disease."

We must reaffirm that the reason for medicine is the PERSON, rather than the reverse.

A hundred years ago medicine had as a primary strategy the need to confront the pestilences that ruled the world. A broadly based counterattack generated much confidence that any future threat could be overcome providing medical science had enough cash in the bank. Sounds logical.

But what if the science is wrong?

John Ioannidis is a Stanford medical colleague. He is a heretic, uttering blasphemy from the front row of the cathedral. His recent Atlantic article, "Lies, Damned Lies, and Medical Science", challenges the grail of medicine. His deep scrutiny of the top medical journals and articles proclaim their lack of credibility. If you can't believe the gospel, what can you believe? The entirety of the sacred science of medicine is suspect. Trust crumbles.

The science should pursue strenuously what the health assurance needs are.

Not what pays.

Yet the Medical Industrial Complex has gorged itself on technology in the hope that a pill or an operation will take care of the problem.

WRONG!

The global health needs now will not yield to technology. They are too personal. The consuming epidemic of chronic disease is grandly susceptible to prevention. With this stark, but only grudgingly acknowledged reality Next Medicine must INSIST on health rather than disease.

Flexner II must mandate that the WHOLE of Medicine become morally and scientifically and economically sound.

Health must pay.

The primary focus must be within the individual, not outside in some money-grubbing enterprise.

This categorical shift in focus is critical. It demands that our lifelong wellbeing is directly the result of decisions made and not made.

Behavior assumes highest priority.

Health is our most important asset.

Take control of it.

Occupy your health!

POST SCRIPT

Winston Churchill marvelously observed, "America is a great country. It invariably gets things right, but only after it has already tried other things first."

Our political attention has been fixed on what happened behind the paneled doors of the United States Supreme Court. Will Mandated Universal Health Insurance emerge intact, or will it be slaughtered by politics?

The bigger issue will arise AFTER Universal Coverage has been initiated.

"Coverage of what?" is now the focus.

Will we continue to shovel mountains of cash and energy and misery into the black hole of current disease medicine?

Or can we change the paradigm to health?

Its fate should represent the will of the people, not that of the financial powers who hold the rudder of the Ship of State.

What if the aspirations of Occupy Medicine are realized?

Then all future generations will genuflect to our era.

www.walterbortz.com

Made in the USA
San Bernardino, CA
10 March 2014